ORLIS

The Concise User Guide Designed for the Treatment and Cure Of Obesity and Used for Weight Loss and Fat Loss in Overweight Adults

ISBN 978-1-716-06191-2

Copyright@2020 By Jarek Rex

COPYRIGHT

All rights reserved. No part of this publication may be reproduced, distributed, or transmitted in any form or by any means, including photocopying, recording, or other electronic or mechanical methods, without the prior written permission of the publisher, except in the case of brief quotations embodied in critical reviews and certain other noncommercial user permitted by copyright law

TABLE OF CONTENT

Chapter 1 4
WHAT IS ORLISTAT AND HOW DOES IT WORK? 4
Doses of Orlistat: 4

CHAPTER 2 8
WHAT ARE SIDE EFFECTS ASSOCIATED WITH USING ORLISTAT? 8

CHAPTER 3 12
WHAT OTHER DRUGS INTERACT WITH ORLISTAT? 12

CHAPTER 4 15
WHAT ARE WARNINGS AND PRECAUTIONS FOR ORLISTAT? 15

CHAPTER 5 23
For what reason is this medicine recommended? 23
How could this medication be utilized? 24

CHAPTER 6 26
Prior to taking orlistat, ... 26
What results can this medicine cause? 31

THE END 39

Chapter 1
WHAT IS ORLISTAT AND HOW DOES IT WORK?

Orlistat is a gastrointestinal lipase inhibitor that works by obstructing osmosis of 25% of the fat in a dinner and is used for weight decrease in overweight adults, 18 years and more settled, when used close by a lessened calorie and low-fat eating routine.

Orlistat is accessible under the accompanying diverse brand names: Alli, and Xenical.

Doses of Orlistat:

Grown-up and Pediatric Dosage Forms and Strengths

Case

60 mg (Alli)

120mg (Xenical)

Stoutness Management

Demonstrated in patients with pretreatment BMI more noteworthy than 30 kg/m², or BMI more prominent than 27 kg/m² in presence of other danger variables or infections (e.g., hypertension, diabetes mellitus, hyperlipidemia)

Grown-up

Rx (Xenical): 120 mg orally at regular intervals with each fat-containing dinner (during or as long as 1 hour after the feast), portions more noteworthy than 120 mg multiple times every day show no extra advantage

Over-the-Counter (OTC) (Alli): Up to 60 mg orally at regular intervals with each fat containing dinner

Kids under 12 years: Safety and adequacy not set up

Kids 12 years and more established:

Remedy (Rx) (Xenical): 120 mg orally at regular intervals with each fat-containing feast (during or as long as 1 hour after the supper), dosages more noteworthy than 120 mg multiple times every day show no extra advantage

Over-the-Counter (OTC) (Alli): Up to 60 mg orally at regular intervals with each fat containing dinner

Simply powerful as an assistant to caloric limitation, expanded active work, and conduct alteration

CHAPTER 2
WHAT ARE SIDE EFFECTS ASSOCIATED WITH USING ORLISTAT?

Normal symptoms of Orlistat include:

Slick spotting on clothing

Opposite symptoms of orlistat include:

Gas (tooting) with release

Greasy/sleek stools

Expanded crap

Fecal incontinence/failure to control defecations

Critical defecations

Free stools

Mud shaded stools

Looseness of the bowels

Rectal torment

Queasiness

Retching

Diminished ingestion of fat solvent nutrients and beta-carotene

Liver disappointment

Oxalate nephropathy

Leukocytoclastic vasculitis

Expanded number of solid discharges

Stomach torment

Shortcoming

Dim pee

Tingling

Loss of craving

Yellowing of the skin or eyes (jaundice)

Issues with your teeth or gums

Cold manifestations (stodgy nose, sniffling, hack, fever, chills, sore throat, influenza indications)

Migraine

Back torment

Skin rash

This archive doesn't contain all conceivable results and others may happen. Check with your doctor for extra data about results.

CHAPTER 3
WHAT OTHER DRUGS INTERACT WITH ORLISTAT?

In the event that your primary care physician has guided you to utilize this prescription, your PCP or drug specialist may as of now know about any conceivable medication collaborations and might be observing you for them. Try not to begin, stop, or change the measurement of any medication prior to checking with your primary care physician, medical care supplier or drug specialist first.

Orlistat has no known serious associations with other various medications.

Orlistat has no known genuine cooperations with other various medications.

Orlistat has moderate associations with in any event 65 unique medications.

Orlistat has mellow connections with in any event 21 distinct medications.

This data doesn't contain every conceivable communication or antagonistic impacts. Thusly, prior to utilizing this item, tell your primary care physician or drug specialist of the multitude of items you use. Keep a rundown of every one of your meds with you, and offer this data with your PCP and drug specialist. Check with your medical services proficient or specialist for extra clinical guidance, or on the off chance that you have wellbeing questions, concerns or for more data about this medication.

CHAPTER 4
WHAT ARE WARNINGS AND PRECAUTIONS FOR ORLISTAT?

Admonitions

This medicine contains orlistat. Try not to take Alli or Xenical on the off chance that you are susceptible to orlistat or any fixings contained in this medication.

Keep far from kids. In the event of excess, get clinical assistance or contact a Poison Control Center right away.

Contraindications

Touchiness

Pregnancy

Persistent malabsorption condition

Cholestasis

Impacts of Drug Abuse

Interpretation content

Alerts

On the off chance that a supper is missed or contains no fat, portion ought to be precluded.

Every day fat admission (30% of calories), carb, and protein ought to be equally conveyed more than 3 fundamental suppers.

Note: Multivitamin supplement (counting nutrients A, D, E, K) is suggested.

Postmarketing reports of serious liver injury with hepatocellular rot or intense hepatic disappointment for certain cases bringing about liver transfer or demise.

History of hyperoxaluria or calcium oxalate nephrolithiasis; instances of oxalate nephrolithiasis and oxalate nephropathy with renal disappointment have been accounted for.

Generous weight reduction can expand danger of cholelithiasis.

Prohibit natural reasons for heftiness (e.g., hypothyroidism), prior to recommending treatment.

May increment gastrointestinal occasions when taking an eating regimen high on fat (more prominent than 30% complete every day calories from fat).

Diabetes mellitus.

Maintain a strategic distance from with anorexia nervosa or bulimia.

Medication association outline:

Cyclosporine: Administer cyclosporine 3 hours after orlistat

Levothyroxine: Administer 4 hours separated; observed for changes in thyroid capacity

Amiodarone oral: A pharmacokinetic study showed decreased amiodarone and desethylamiodarone fundamental openness when coadministered with orlistat

Antiepileptic drugs (AEDs): Convulsions detailed with coadministration of AEDs and orlistat; screen serum AED levels

Antiretroviral drugs: Loss of virological control has been accounted for in HIV-contaminated patients taking orlistat correspondingly with antiretroviral drugs; HIV RNA levels ought to be oftentimes checked in patients taking orlistat and antiretroviral drugs; if HIV viral burden builds, end orlistat

Warfarin

Nutrient K ingestion might be diminished with orlistat

Reports of diminished prothrombin, expanded INR, and uneven anticoagulant treatment bringing about difference in hemostatic boundaries have been with coadministration of orlistat and anticoagulants

Patients on ongoing stable dosages of warfarin or different anticoagulants who are recommended orlistat ought to be observed intently for coagulation boundaries changes

Nutrient enhancements

Orlistat may diminish assimilation of some fat-dissolvable nutrients and beta-carotene

Train patient to take a multivitamin containing fat-solvent nutrients to guarantee sufficient sustenance

Take nutrient enhancement in any event 2 hours prior or subsequent to taking orlistat, for example, at sleep time

Pregnancy and Lactation

Try not to utilize orlistat in pregnancy. The dangers included exceed expected advantages. More secure choices exist. Weight reduction offers no expected advantage to a pregnant lady and may bring about fetal mischief. A base weight acquire, and no weight reduction, is as of now suggested for every single pregnant lady, including the individuals who are as of now overweight or large.

It isn't known whether orlistat is circulated in bosom milk. Orlistat isn't suggested for use while breastfeeding.

CHAPTER 5
For what reason is this medicine recommended?

Orlistat (remedy and nonprescription) is utilized with an individualized low-calorie, low-fat eating routine and exercise program to assist individuals with shedding pounds. Remedy orlistat is utilized in overweight individuals who may likewise have hypertension, diabetes, elevated cholesterol, or coronary illness. Orlistat is likewise utilized after weight reduction to help individuals hold back from restoring that weight. Orlistat is in a class of meds called lipase inhibitors. It works by forestalling a portion of the fat in nourishments eaten from being caught up in the digestive organs. This unabsorbed fat is then eliminated from the body in the stool.

How could this medication be utilized?

Orlistat comes as a case and a nonprescription container to take by mouth. It is typically required three times each day with every primary dinner that contains fat. Take orlistat during a supper or as long as 1 hour after a feast. In the event that a feast is missed or doesn't have fat, you may skirt your portion. Follow the headings on your medicine mark or the bundle name cautiously, and ask your primary care physician or drug specialist to clarify any part you don't comprehend. Take orlistat precisely as coordinated. Try not to take pretty much of it or take it more regularly than endorsed by your primary care physician or expressed on the bundle.

Request your drug specialist or specialist for a duplicate from the maker's data for the patient if orlistat is recommended for you. For extra data about the nonprescription item, visit http://www.MyAlli.com.

Different utilizations for this medication

This drug is now and then endorsed for different utilizations; ask your primary care physician or drug specialist for more data.

CHAPTER 6
Prior to taking orlistat,

tell your PCP and drug specialist in the event that you are oversensitive to orlistat or some other prescriptions.

converse with your primary care physician on the off chance that you are taking drugs that stifle the insusceptible framework, for example, cyclosporine (Neoral, Sandimmune). On the off chance that you are taking cyclosporine (Neoral, Sandimmune), take it 2 hours prior or 2 hours after orlistat.

mention to your PCP and drug specialist what remedy and nonprescription, nutrients, wholesome enhancements, and home grown items you are taking or plan to take. Make certain to specify any of the accompanying: anticoagulants ("blood thinners, for example, warfarin (Coumadin); drugs for diabetes, for example, glipizide (Glucotrol), glyburide (DiaBeta, Dynase, Micronase), metformin (Glucophage), and insulin; meds to control circulatory strain; meds for thyroid illness; and some other meds for weight reduction.

tell your primary care physician in the event that you have in the event that you have had an organ relocate or on the off chance that you have cholestasis (condition in which the progression of bile from the liver is hindered) or malabsorption disorder (issues engrossing food). Your PCP will likely disclose to you not to take orlistat.

tell your PCP in the event that you have or have at any point had a dietary issue, for example, anorexia nervosa or bulimia, diabetes, kidney stones, pancreatitis (irritation or growing of the pancreas), or gallbladder or thyroid sickness.

tell your PCP in the event that you are pregnant, plan to get pregnant, or are bosom taking care of. Try not to take orlistat on the off chance that you are pregnant or bosom taking care of.

What exceptional dietary directions would it be a good idea for me to follow?

Follow the eating routine program your primary care physician has given you. You ought to equally isolate the measure of every day fat, sugars, and protein you eat more than three primary suppers. On the off chance that you take orlistat with an eating routine high in fat (an eating regimen with over 30% of the absolute every day calories from fat), or with one supper high in fat, you are bound to encounter results from the drug.

While you are taking orlistat, you ought to evade nourishments that have over 30% fat. Peruse the marks on all the food sources you purchase. When eating meat, poultry (chicken) or fish, eat just 2 or 3 ounces (55 or 85 grams) (about the size of a deck of cards) for a serving. Pick lean cuts of meat and eliminate the skin from poultry. Top off your dinner plate with more grains, organic products, and vegetables. Supplant entire milk items with nonfat or 1% milk and decreased or low-fat dairy things. Cook with less fat. Utilize vegetable oil shower when cooking. Plate of mixed greens dressings; many heated things; and prepackaged, prepared, and quick nourishments are typically high in fat. Utilize the low-or nonfat adaptations of these food sources and additionally cut back on serving sizes. When eating out, ask how nourishments are arranged and demand that they be set up with almost no additional fat.

Orlistat blocks your body's assimilation of some fat-dissolvable nutrients and beta carotene. Thusly, when you use orlistat you should take an every day multivitamin that contains nutrients A, D, E, K, and beta-carotene. Peruse the name to discover a multivitamin item that contains these nutrients. Take the multivitamin once every day, 2 hours prior or 2 hours subsequent to taking orlistat, or take the multivitamin at sleep time. Ask your PCP or drug specialist any inquiries you may have about taking a multivitamin while you are taking orlistat.

How would it be a good idea for me to respond on the off chance that I fail to remember a portion?

Accept the missed portion when you recollect it except if it is over 1 hour since you ate a primary dinner. In the event that it is longer than 1 hour since you ate a principle feast, skirt the missed portion and proceed on your ordinary dosing plan.

What results can this medicine cause?

Orlistat may cause results. The most widely recognized symptom of orlistat is changes in solid discharge (BM) propensities. This by and large happens during the primary long stretches of treatment; nonetheless, it might proceed all through your utilization of orlistat. Tell your PCP if any of these manifestations are serious or don't disappear:

slick spotting on clothing or on dress

gas with slick spotting

dire need to have a solid discharge

free stools

slick or greasy stools

expanded number of defecations

trouble controlling defecations

torment or inconvenience in the rectum (base)

stomach torment

unpredictable feminine periods

cerebral pain

uneasiness

Some results can be not kidding. In the event that you experience any of these indications, call your PCP right away:

hives

rash

tingling

trouble breathing or gulping

serious or constant stomach torment

exorbitant sluggishness or shortcoming

queasiness

spewing

loss of craving

yellowing of the skin or eyes

dim hued pee

light-hued stools

On the off chance that you experience a genuine result, you or your primary care physician may send a report to the Food and Drug Administration's (FDA) MedWatch Adverse Event Reporting program on the web (http://www.fda.gov/Safety/MedWatch) or by telephone (1-800-332-1088).

Orlistat may cause opposite results. Call your PCP in the event that you have any irregular issues during your treatment with orlistat.

A few people who took orlistat created serious liver harm. There isn't sufficient data to tell whether the liver harm was brought about by orlistat. Converse with your primary care physician about the dangers of taking orlistat.

What would it be a good idea for me to think about capacity and removal of this prescription?

Store it at room temperature and away from abundance heat, dampness (not in the washroom), and light.

Unneeded prescriptions ought to be discarded in unique manners to guarantee that pets, kids, and others can't burn-through them.

All things considered, the most ideal approach to discard your drug is through a medication reclaim program. Converse with your drug specialist or contact your nearby trash/reusing division to find out about reclaim programs locally. See the FDA's Safe Disposal of Medicines site (http://goo.gl/c4Rm4p) for more data on the off chance that you don't approach a reclaim program.

It is essential to keep all prescription far out and reach of youngsters as numerous compartments, (for example, week by week pill minders and those for eye drops, creams, patches

To shield small kids from harming, consistently lock security covers and promptly place the drug in a protected area – one that is up into the clouds and out of their sight and reach.

If there should arise an occurrence of crisis/glut

If there should arise an occurrence of excess, call the toxin control helpline at 1-800-222-1222. Data is likewise accessible online at https://www.poisonhelp.org/help. In the event that the casualty has imploded, had a seizure, experiences difficulty breathing, or can't be stirred, promptly call crisis administrations at 911.

You ought to likewise follow a program of ordinary active work or exercise while you are taking orlistat. Notwithstanding, before you start any new movement or exercise program, talk with your PCP or medical services proficient.

Try not to let any other person take your physician recommended prescription.

It is significant for you to keep a composed rundown of the entirety of the solution and nonprescription (over-the-counter) drugs you are taking, just as any items, for example, nutrients, minerals, or other dietary enhancements.

THE END

CPSIA information can be obtained
at www.ICGtesting.com
Printed in the USA
LVHW011750160621
690401LV00014B/1272